Sirtfood Diet Meal Prep

Discover Surprisingly Healthy Meals to Lose 7 pounds in only 7 days!

Bree Osborne

Well-Belly Press

GREEN JUICES 6

Celery, Carrot & Orange Juice 7

Orange & Kale Juice 8

Apple, Carrot & Celery Juice 9

Apple, Kale & Parsley Juice 10

Apple, Cucumber & Celery Juice 11

Apple & Celery Juice 12

Kale & Apple Juice 13

Kale & Celery Juice 14

Apple, Orange & Broccoli Juice 15

Kale, Carrot & Fruit Juice 16

Kale, Celery, Apple & Orange Juice 17

Kale, Celery & Pear Juice 18

Green Fruit Juice 19

Matcha, Apple & Greens Juice 20

Parsley Green Juice 21

Spinach & Apple Juice 22

Parsley Creamy Juice 23

Parsley Green Juice 24

Mix Green Juice 25

Rosemary Green Juice 26

Cilantro & Lettuce Juice 27

Cucumber Creamy Juice 28

Kale & Kiwi Juice 29

Broccoli Green Juice 30

Berries Green Juice 31

Fluffy Avocado Juice 32

Broccoli Apple Juice 33

Rocket Green Juice 34

Swiss Chard Green Juice 35

Kale Green Juice 36

Arugula leaves Juice 37

BREAKFAST 38

Spinach Porridge 39

Italian Spinach Tofu Omelet 40

Tofu & Arugula Toast 41

Breakfast Tofu Scramble 42

Buckwheat& walnuts Pancakes..43

Breakfast Tofu Waffles...44

Savory Buckwheat Porridge..45

French Toast with Berries...46

Buckwheat Crepe with Berries..47

Kiwi & Apple Porridge..48

Strawberry Smoothie Bowl...49

Berries Pancakes..50

Walnut Cream Parfait...51

Chocolate Pancakes...52

Tofu & Spinach Muffins...53

Turmeric Tofu Toast...54

Apple Bread Loaf..55

Zucchini Tots...56

Tofu & Berries Waffles..57

Chocolate Pudding...58

Cinnamon & Walnut Tea...59

Apple Porridge...60

Kale Omelet...61

Tofu & Kale Toast...62

Tofu Scramble..63

Buckwheat Pancakes..64

Waffle Sandwich...65

Buckwheat Porridge..66

Toast with Caramelized Apple...67

MAIN MEALS..68

Creamy Spinach Curry..69

Broccoli Olives Pizza..70

Buffalo Broccoli Bites...71

Spinach Soup...72

Chili Tofu...73

Spicy Spinach Fillet..74

Broccoli Patties..75

Spinach & Tofu Pizza..76

Broccoli Flatbread Pizza...77

Turmeric Spinach Patties..78

Stir Fried Broccoli & Tofu..79

Wilted Spinach with Onion..80

Broccoli with Garlic sauce..81

Hot & Sour Spinach 82

Spinach & Tofu Curry 83

Sardine Puttanesca Spaghetti 84

Tofu Power Bowls 85

Superfood Bibimbap With Crispy Tofu............................ 87

Spicy Tofu Kale Wraps...89

Tofu Burritos 90

Asian Garlic Tofu...92

Tofu Burritos Recipe 2...94

Hot & Sour Soup..96

Tofu & Avocado Spring Rolls.. 97

Simple Tofu Quiche..99

Barbecued Waffle Iron Tofu...101

Cauliflower Mac 'n' Cheese 102

Beans & Broccolini...104

Chicken Stew..105

Baked Chicken with Salad 106

Lamb Chops with Salad 108

Flank Steak with Salad 110

Glazed Flank Steak..111

Apple & Walnuts Cake 114

Baked Walnut Brownies 115

Coco & Walnuts Smoothie...116

Walnut Cream Cake.. 117

Walnuts Bits...118

Walnuts Bites Muffins..119

Buckwheat Cinnamon Buns 120

GREEN JUICES

Celery, Carrot & Orange Juice

Preparation time: 10 min

Serves: 2

What you need:
- 4 celery stalks with leaves
- 3 medium carrots, peeled and chopped
- **2** oranges, peeled and sectioned
- **1** tablespoon fresh ginger, peeled

Method:
1. Place all ingredients in a high-powered blender and pulse until well combined.
2. Through a fine mesh strainer, strain the juice and transfer it into two glasses.
3. Serve immediately.

Per serving:
Calories Per **Serves:**, 181 kcal, 1.72 g Fat, 39.64 g Total Carbs, 10.41 g Protein, 12.2 g Fiber

Orange & Kale Juice

Preparation time: 10 min

Serves: 2

What you need:
- 4 large oranges, peeled and sectioned
- **2** bunches fresh kale

Method:
1. Put all ingredients in a juicer and extract the juice according to the manufacturer's instructions.
2. Pour into two glasses and serve immediately.

Per serving:
Calories Per **Serves:**, 181 kcal, 0.4 g Fat, 57 g Total Carbs, 10.41 g Protein, 7 g Fiber

Apple, Carrot & Celery Juice

Preparation time: 10 min

Serves: 2

What you need:

- 5 carrots, peeled and chopped
- **1** large apple, cored and chopped
- **2** celery stalks
- **1** (½-inch) piece fresh ginger, peeled and chopped
- ½ of lemon

Method:

1. Put all ingredients in a juicer and extract the juice according to the manufacturer's instructions.
2. Pour into two glasses and serve immediately.

Per serving:

Calories Per **Serves:**, 126 kcal, 0.3 g Fat, 31 g Total Carbs, 1 g Protein, 6 g Fiber

Apple, Kale & Parsley Juice

Preparation time: 10 min

Serves: 2

What you need:

- **2** large green apples, cored and sliced
- 4 cups fresh kale leaves
- 4 tablespoons fresh parsley leaves
- **1** tablespoon fresh ginger, peeled
- **1** lemon, peeled
- ½ cup filtered water
- Pinch of salt

Method:

1. Place all ingredients in a high-powered blender and pulse until well combined.
2. Through a fine mesh strainer, strain the juice and transfer it into two glasses.
3. Serve immediately.

Per serving:

Calories Per **Serves:**, 197 kcal, 0.7 g Fat, 48 g Total Carbs, 5 g Protein, 8 g Fiber

Apple, Cucumber & Celery Juice

Preparation time: 10 min

Serves: 2

What you need:

- 3 large apples, cored and sliced
- **2** large cucumbers, sliced
- 4 celery stalks
- **1 (1**-inch) piece fresh ginger, peeled
- **1** lemon, peeled

Method:

1. Put all ingredients in a juicer and extract the juice according to the manufacturer's instructions.
2. Pour into two glasses and serve immediately.

Per serving:

Calories Per **Serves:**, 230 kcal, 1 g Fat, 59 g Total Carbs, 3 g Protein, 10 g Fiber

Apple & Celery Juice

Preparation time: 10 min

Serves: 2

What you need:

- 4 large green apples, cored and sliced
- 4 celery stalks
- **1** lemon, peeled

Method:

1. Put all ingredients in a juicer and extract the juice according to the manufacturer's instructions.
2. Pour into two glasses and serve immediately.

Per serving:

Calories Per **Serves:**, 240 kcal, 0.9 g Fat, 63 g Total Carbs, 1 g Protein, 11 g Fiber

Kale & Apple Juice

Preparation time: 10 min

Serves: 2

What you need:
- 3 large green apples, cored and sliced
- 4 cups fresh kale leaves
- **2** tablespoons fresh lemon juice
- ½ cup filtered water

Method:
1. Put all ingredients in a juicer and extract the juice according to the manufacturer's instructions.
2. Pour into two glasses and serve immediately.

Per serving:
Calories Per **Serves:**, 244 kcal, 0.7 g Fat, 60 g Total Carbs, 5 g Protein, 10 g Fiber

Kale & Celery Juice

Preparation time: 10 min

Serves: 2

What you need:
- 4 celery stalks
- 5 cups fresh kale leaves
- **1** (½-inch) piece fresh ginger, peeled
- **1** lime, halved

Method:
1. Put all ingredients in a juicer and extract the juice according to the manufacturer's instructions.
2. Pour into two glasses and serve immediately.

Per serving:
Calories Per **Serves:**, 91 kcal, 0.1 g Fat, 19 g Total Carbs, 5 g Protein, 3 g Fiber

Apple, Orange & Broccoli Juice

Preparation time: 10 min

Serves: 2

What you need:

- **2** broccoli stalks, chopped
- **2** large green apples, cored and sliced
- 3 large oranges, peeled and sectioned
- 4 tablespoons fresh parsley

Method:

1. Put all ingredients in a juicer and extract the juice according to the manufacturer's instructions.
2. Pour into two glasses and serve immediately.

Per serving:

Calories Per **Serves:**, 254 kcal, 0.8 g Fat, 64 g Total Carbs, 3 g Protein, 12 g Fiber

Kale, Carrot & Fruit Juice

Preparation time: 10 min

Serves: 2

What you need:
- 3 cups fresh kale
- **2** large apples, cored and sliced
- **2** medium carrots, peeled and chopped
- **2** medium grapefruit, peeled and sectioned
- **1** teaspoon fresh lemon juice

Method:
1. Put all ingredients in a juicer and extract the juice according to the manufacturer's instructions.
2. Pour into two glasses and serve immediately.

Per serving:
Calories Per **Serves:**, 232 kcal, 0 g Fat, 57g Total Carbs, 4 g Protein, 9 g Fiber

Kale, Celery, Apple & Orange Juice

Preparation time: 10 min

Serves: 2

What you need:

- 3 cups fresh kale, chopped
- **2** large celery stalks, chopped
- **2** large green apples, cored and sliced
- **1** large orange, peeled and sectioned
- **1** tablespoon fresh lime juice
- **1** tablespoon fresh lemon juice

Method:

1. Put all ingredients in a juicer and extract the juice according to the manufacturer's instructions.
2. Pour into two glasses and serve immediately.

Per serving:

Calories Per **Serves:**, 214 kcal, 0.1 g Fat, 52 g Total Carbs, 4 g Protein, 9 g Fiber

Kale, Celery & Pear Juice

Preparation time: 10 min

Serves: 2

What you need:
- 6 pears, cored and chopped
- 3 celery stalks
- 3 cups fresh kale
- **2** tablespoons fresh parsley

Method:
1. Put all ingredients in a juicer and extract the juice according to the manufacturer's instructions.
2. Pour into two glasses and serve immediately.

Per serving:

Calories Per **Serves:**, 209 kcal, 0.9g Fat, 50 g Total Carbs, 5 g Protein, 15 g Fiber

Green Fruit Juice

Preparation time: 10 min

Serves: 2

What you need:
- 3 large kiwis, peeled and chopped
- **2** large green apples, cored and sliced
- **2** cups seedless green grapes
- **2** teaspoons fresh lime juice

Method:
1. Put all ingredients in a juicer and extract the juice according to the manufacturer's instructions.
2. Pour into two glasses and serve immediately.

Per serving:
Calories Per **Serves:**, 265 kcal, 0.6g Fat, 68 g Total Carbs, 1 g Protein, 9 g Fiber

Matcha, Apple & Greens Juice

Preparation time: 10 min

Serves: 2

What you need:

- 5 ounces fresh kale
- **2** ounces fresh arugula
- ¼ cup fresh parsley
- 4 celery stalks
- **1** green apple, cored and chopped
- **1 (1**-inch) piece fresh ginger, peeled
- **1** lemon, peeled
- ½ teaspoon matcha green tea

Method:

1. Put all ingredients in a juicer and extract the juice according to the manufacturer's instructions.
2. Pour into two glasses and serve immediately.

Per serving:

Calories Per **Serves:**, 113 kcal, 0.6 g Fat, 26 g Total Carbs, 3 g Protein, 5 g Fiber

Parsley Green Juice

Preparation time: 10 min

Serves: 1
What you need:

- 1 bunch parsley
- 1 kiwi fruit
- 1 cucumber
- 1 apple
- half a lemon, juiced
- 1 tsp. matcha green tea

Method:

1. Put parsley, apple, cucumber, and kiwi fruit in an electric juicer and extract the juice.
2. Pour the juice into a glass and mix matcha, lemon juice with a fork.
3. Once the matcha tea powder is mixed in juice add some water.
4. Pour some ice on top.
5. Enjoy!

Per serving:

Calories Per **Serves:**, 181 kcal, 1.72 g Fat, 39.64 g Total Carbs, 10.41 g Protein, 12.2 g Fiber

Spinach & Apple Juice

Preparation time: 10 min

Serves: 1
What you need:

- 1 bunch baby spinach
- 1 apple
- ¼ cup mixed berries
- 1/8 tsp. ginger
- half a lemon, juiced
- 1 tsp. matcha green tea

Method:

1. Put spinach, apple, and berries in an electric juicer and extract the juice.
2. Pour the juice into a glass and mix matcha, lemon juice with a fork.
3. Once the matcha tea powder is mixed in juice add some water.
4. Pour some ice on top.
5. Enjoy!

Per serving:

Calories Per **Serves:**, 121 kcal, 0.49 g Fat, 32.2 g Total Carbs, 0.85 g Protein, 5.3 g Fiber

Parsley Creamy Juice

Preparation time: 10 min

Serves: 1

What you need:

- 1 bunch parsley
- 1 green apple
- 1 cup broccoli
- 1/8 tsp ginger
- ¼ cup walnut milk
- half a lemon, juiced
- 1 tsp. matcha green tea

Method:

1. Put parsley, apple, broccoli, and ginger in an electric juicer and extract the juice.
2. Pour the juice into a glass and mix matcha, lemon juice with a fork.
3. Once the matcha tea powder is mixed in juice add some water and milk
4. Pour some ice on top.
5. Enjoy!

Per serving:

Calories Per **Serves:**, 187 kcal, 1.89 g Fat, 40.33 g Total Carbs, 11.56 g Protein, 13 g Fiber

Parsley Green Juice

Preparation time: 10 min

Serves: 1

What you need:

- 1 bunch parsley leaves
- 2 stalk celery
- 1 apple
- half a lemon, juiced
- 1 tsp. matcha green tea

Method:

1. Put parsley, apple, and celery in an electric juicer and extract the juice.
2. Pour the juice into a glass and mix matcha, lemon juice with a fork.
3. Once the matcha tea powder is mixed in juice add some water.
4. Pour some ice on top.
5. Enjoy!

Per serving:

 Calories Per Serves:, 118 kcal, 0.55 g Fat, 3o.07 g Total Carbs, 1.33 g Protein, 6.2 g Fiber

Mix Green Juice

Preparation time: 10 min

Serves: 1

What you need:

- 1 bunch spinach leaves
- 1 apple
- 1 cucumber
- half a lemon, juiced
- 1 tsp. matcha green tea

Method:

1. Put spinach, apple, cucumber, and kiwi fruit in an electric juicer and extract the juice.
2. Pour the juice into a glass and mix matcha, lemon juice with a fork.
3. Once the matcha tea powder is mixed in juice add some water.
4. Pour some ice on top.
5. Enjoy!

Per serving:

Calories Per Serves:, 146 kcal, 1.16 g Fat, 33.93 g Total Carbs, 3.53 g Protein, 7.8 g Fiber

Rosemary Green Juice

Preparation time: 10 min

Serves: 1

What you need:

- 2 bunch baby spinach
- 1 cup chopped rosemary
- 1 apple
- 1 cucumber
- ¼ cup walnut milk
- half a lemon, juiced
- 1 tsp. matcha green tea

Method:

1. Put spinach, rosemary, apple, cucumber in an electric juicer and extract the juice.
2. Pour the juice into a glass and mix matcha, lemon juice with a fork.
3. Once the matcha tea powder is mixed in juice add some water and walnut milk.
4. Pour some ice on top.
5. Enjoy!

Per serving:

Calories Per **Serves:**, 171 kcal, 1.67 g Fat, 39.53 g Total Carbs, 6.54 g Protein, 9.8 g Fiber

Cilantro & Lettuce Juice

Preparation time: 10 min

Serves: 1
What you need:

- 1 bunch cilantro leaves
- 4-5 lettuce leaves
- 1 apple
- half a lemon, juiced
- 1 tsp. matcha green tea

Method:

1. Put cilantro, apple, and lettuce in an electric juicer and extract the juice.
2. Pour the juice into a glass and mix matcha, lemon juice with a fork.
3. Once the matcha tea powder is mixed in juice add some water.
4. Pour some ice on top.
5. Enjoy!

Per serving:

Calories Per **Serves:**, 178 kcal, 1.69 g Fat, 39.13 g Total Carbs, 10.29 g Protein, 11.9 g Fiber

Cucumber Creamy Juice

Preparation time: 10 min

Serves: 19
What you need:

- 2 cucumbers
- 1 green apple
- ¼ cup walnut milk
- half a lemon, juiced
- 1 tsp. matcha green tea

Method:

1. Put cucumber, apple in an electric juicer and extract the juice.
2. Pour the juice into a glass and mix matcha, lemon juice with a fork.
3. Once the matcha tea powder is mixed in juice add some water and walnut milk.
4. Pour some ice on top.
5. Enjoy!

Per serving:

Calories Per **Serves:**, 124 kcal, 0.69 g Fat, 31.13 g Total Carbs, 1.75 g Protein, 5.8 g Fiber

Kale & Kiwi Juice

Preparation time: 10 min

Serves: 1
What you need:

- 1 bunch kale
- ½ cup soy milk
- 1 kiwi fruit
- half a medium green apple
- half a lemon, juiced
- 1 tsp. matcha green tea

Method:

1. Put kale and kiwi fruit in an electric juicer and extract the juice.
2. Pour the juice into a glass and mix matcha, lemon juice with a fork.
3. Once the matcha tea powder is mixed in juice add some water and soy milk.
4. Pour some ice on top.
5. Enjoy!

Per serving:

Calories Per **Serves:**, 185 kcal, 3.35 g Fat, 32.68 g Total Carbs, 13.28 g Protein, 10 g Fiber

Broccoli Green Juice

Preparation time: 10 min

Serves: 1
What you need:

- 1 head broccoli
- 1 bunch spinach leaves
- 1 apple
- half a lemon, juiced
- 1 tsp. matcha green tea

Method:

1. Put broccoli, spinach, apple in an electric juicer and extract the juice.
2. Pour the juice into a glass and mix matcha, lemon juice with a fork.
3. Once the matcha tea powder is mixed in juice add some water.
4. Pour some ice on top.
5. Enjoy!

Per serving:
Calories Per **Serves:**, 124 kcal, 0.87 g Fat, 31.9 g Total Carbs, 2.47 g Protein, 6.7 g Fiber

Berries Green Juice

Preparation time: 10 min

Serves: 1

What you need:

- 1 bunch mint leaves
- 1 apple
- large stalks green celery, including leaves
- 1 cup mixed berries
- half a lemon, juiced
- 1 tsp. matcha green tea

Method:

1. Put mint leaves, apple, celery, and berries in an electric juicer and extract the juice.
2. Pour the juice into a glass and mix matcha, lemon juice with a fork.
3. Once the matcha tea powder is mixed in juice add some water.
4. Pour some ice on top.
5. Enjoy!

Per serving:

Calories Per **Serves:**, 181 kcal, 1.72 g Fat, 39.64 g Total Carbs, 10.41 g Protein, 12.2 g Fiber

Fluffy Avocado Juice

Preparation time: 10 min

Serves: 1
What you need:

- 1 head broccoli
- 1 apple
- ¼ cup avocado
- 1/8 tsp. ginger
- half a lemon, juiced
- 1 tsp. matcha green tea

Method:

1. Put broccoli, apple, avocado, and ginger in an electric juicer and extract the juice.
2. Pour the juice into a glass and mix matcha, lemon juice with a fork.
3. Once the matcha tea powder is mixed in juice add some water.
4. Pour some ice on top.
5. Enjoy!

Per serving:

Calories Per **Serves:**, 121 kcal, 0.49 g Fat, 32.2 g Total Carbs, 0.85 g Protein, 5.3 g Fiber

Broccoli Apple Juice

Preparation time: 10 min

Serves: 1
What you need:

- 1 bunch spinach
- 1 apple
- 1 cup broccoli
- 1/8 tsp ginger
- half a lemon, juiced
- 1 tsp. matcha green tea

Method:

1. Put spinach, apple, broccoli, and ginger in an electric juicer and extract the juice.
2. Pour the juice into a glass and mix matcha, lemon juice with a fork.
3. Once the matcha tea powder is mixed in juice add some water.
4. Pour some ice on top.
5. Enjoy!

Per serving:

Calories Per **Serves:**, 187 kcal, 1.89 g Fat, 40.33 g Total Carbs, 11.56 g Protein, 13 g Fiber

Rocket Green Juice

Preparation time: 10 min

Serves: 1

What you need:

- 1 rocket leaves
- 1 apple
- 1 cucumber
- half a lemon, juiced
- 1 tsp. matcha green tea

Method:

1. Put rocket leaves, apples, and cucumber in an electric juicer and extract the juice.
2. Pour the juice into a glass and mix matcha and lemon juice with a fork.
3. Once the matcha tea powder is mixed in juice, add some water.
4. Pour some ice on top.
5. Enjoy!

Per serving:

Calories Per **Serves:**, 146 kcal, 1.16 g Fat, 33.93 g Total Carbs, 3.53 g Protein, 7.8 g Fiber

Swiss Chard Green Juice

Preparation time: 10 min

Serves: 1
What you need:

- 1 bunch swiss chard leaves
- 1 apple
- half a lemon, juiced
- 1 tsp. matcha green tea

Method:

1. Put Swiss chard leaves, apple in an electric juicer and extract the juice.
2. Pour the juice into a glass and mix matcha, lemon juice with a fork.
3. Once the matcha tea powder is mixed in juice add some water.
4. Pour some ice on top.
5. Enjoy!

Per serving:

Calories Per **Serves:**, 118 kcal, 0.55 g Fat, 3o.07 g Total Carbs, 1.33 g Protein, 6.2 g Fiber

Kale Green Juice

Preparation time: 10 min

Serves: 1
What you need:

- 2 bunch kale
- 1 apple
- 2 stalk celery with leaves
- half a lemon, juiced
- 1 tsp. matcha green tea

Method:

1. Put kale, apple, celery in electric juice and extract the juice.
2. Pour the juice into a glass and mix in matcha and lemon juice with a fork.
3. Once the matcha tea powder is mixed in juice add some water.
4. Pour some ice on top.
5. Enjoy!

Per serving:

Calories Per **Serves:**, 171 kcal, 1.67 g Fat, 39.53 g Total Carbs, 6.54 g Protein, 9.8 g Fiber

Arugula leaves Juice

Preparation time: 10 min

Serves: 1

What you need:

- 1 bunch arugula leaves
- 1 apple
- half a lemon, juiced
- 1 tsp. matcha green tea

Method:

1. Put arugula leaves, apple, in electric juice and extract the juice.
2. Pour the juice into a glass and mix matcha, lemon juice with a fork.
3. Once the matcha tea powder is mixed in juice add some water.
4. Pour some ice on top.
5. Enjoy!

Per serving:

Calories Per **Serves:**, 178 kcal, 1.69 g Fat, 39.13 g Total Carbs, 10.29 g Protein, 11.9 g

Fiber

BREAKFAST

Spinach Porridge

Preparation time: 10 Min

Serves: 2

What you need:

- 2 bunch baby spinach, chopped
- 2 cups walnut milk
- 1 tsp. cinnamon
- 2 tsp. dates syrup

Topping

- Blueberries
- Chia seeds
- Chopped walnuts

Method:

1. Mix all porridge Ingredients in blender.
2. Pour porridge in bowl.
3. Top with blueberries, baby spinach, chia seeds, and chopped walnuts.
4. Serve and enjoy!

Per serving:

Calories Per **Serves:**, 227 kcal, 7.04 g Fat, 36.45 g Total Carbs, 6.95 g Protein, 4.3 g Fiber

Italian Spinach Tofu Omelet

Preparation time: 20 min

Serves: 2

What you need:
- 2 cups baby spinach, finely chopped
- 1 cup, chopped onion
- 1 cup tofu.
- ¼ cup water
- salt & pepper to taste
- 1 tsp. paprika powder
- 1 tsp. oregano
- olive oil for frying

Method:
1. Blend tofu, salt, pepper, oregano, and paprika in a blender until smooth.
2. Add water slowly in the mixture to make a thick batter.
3. Place a frying pan over medium heat and grease with olive oil.
4. Sautee spinach in pan and cook for 4-5 minutes.
5. Pour tofu mixture in skillet and spread it evenly.
6. Once cooked, flip and cook for another 2-3 minutes.
7. Once the omelet is cooked remove it from heat.
8. Serve hot.
9. Enjoy!

Per serving:
Calories Per **Serves:**, 283 kcal, 3.02 g Fat, 57.39 g Total Carbs, 14.52 g Protein, 12.5 g Fiber

Tofu & Arugula Toast

Preparation time: 10 min

Serves: 4

What you need:

- sea salt and black pepper
- 1 tsp. sesame seeds
- 1/4 cup guacamole
- 8 oz. tofu, firm and drained
- 4 slices buckwheat bread
- 1 tbsp. olive oil

Method:

1. Heat olive oil in pan over medium heat, once the oil is hot, add tofu, fry until golden brown from all sides.
2. Toast bread on a heated griddle for 2-3 minutes per side.
3. Spread guacamole on each bread slice and arrange on a plate.
4. Arrange tofu on bread slice with arugula.
5. Drizzle sesame seeds.
6. Serve and enjoy!

Per serving:

Calories Per **Serves:**, 216 kcal, 17.36 g Fat, 8.43 g Total Carbs, 10.45 g Protein, 3.5 g Fiber

Breakfast Tofu Scramble

Preparation time: 20 min

Serves: 2
What you need:

- 1 tablespoon olive oil
- 16 oz. block firm tofu
- 1 teaspoon salt
- 1/4 teaspoon turmeric
- 1/4 teaspoon garlic powder
- 2 tablespoons soy milk

Serving

- 1 buckwheat slice
- Bell pepper.
- Baby spinach leaves

Method:

1. Heat the olive oil in a pan over medium heat.
2. Crumble the block of tofu right in the pan, with a potato masher or a fork.
3. Cook & stir for 3-4 minutes until the water from the tofu is dried.
4. Add salt, turmeric, and garlic powder.
5. Cook and stir for another 5 minutes.
6. Pour the milk into the pan, and stir to mix. Serve immediately with baby spinach, sauté veggies, and buckwheat leaves.
7. Enjoy!

Per serving:
Calories Per **Serves:**, 208 kcal, 15.44 g Fat, 5.45g Total Carbs, 15.2 g Protein, 0.6 g Fiber

Buckwheat& walnuts Pancakes

Preparation time: 20 min

Serves: 4
What you need:

- 1 cup buckwheat flour
- 2 tbsps. dates syrup
- 1 cup soya milk
- 1 tbsps. olive oil
- 2 tablespoons walnut chopped

Method:

1. Mix all pancake ingredients in a bowl.
2. Heat oil in pan over medium heat. Once the oil is hot pour ¼ cup pancake batter and spread evenly.
3. Cook for 2-3 minutes until golden brown.
4. Flip and cook again.
5. Once cooked remove from heat.
6. Serve with walnuts and dates syrup on top.
7. Enjoy!

Per serving:

Calories Per **Serves:**, 197 kcal, 3.92 g Fat, 35.68 g Total Carbs, 7.73 g Protein, 4.43g Fiber

Breakfast Tofu Waffles

Preparation time: 10 min

Serves: 4

What you need:

- 1 cup tofu
- 2 teaspoons baking powder
- 1 teaspoon baking soda
- 1/4 teaspoon salt
- 1/4 teaspoon cinnamon
- 1 1/2 cups soy milk,
- 1 tablespoon apple cider vinegar
- 1/8 cup olive oil

Serving

- Fresh berries
- Walnut cream
- Chopped walnut

Method:

1. Mix all waffle ingredients in an electric blender until well incorporated.
2. Preheat a waffle iron and lightly grease with cooking spray.
3. Cook waffles according to the manufacturer's instructions.
4. Serve with fresh berries, walnut cream, and chopped walnut.
5. Enjoy!

Per serving:

Calories Per **Serves:**, 260 kcal, 10.27 g Fat, 38.37 g Total Carbs, 7.16 g Protein, 4.7 g Fiber

Savory Buckwheat Porridge

Preparation time: 10 min

Serves: 4

What you need:

- 1 cup buckwheat groats
- 3 cups water
- 1 tablespoon walnut butter
- ½ tablespoon salt
- ½ cup soya milk
- 1 pinch turmeric
- 1 pinch oregano

Method:

1. In a saucepan bring water to boil.
2. Add buckwheat groats and cook d=covered until cooked through.
3. Turn off heat, add the salt, turmeric, and oregano.
4. Mix well.
5. You can add chopped veggies of your choice.
6. Serve and enjoy!

Per serving:

Calories Per **Serves:**, 188 kcal, 4.6 g Fat, 33.56 g Total Carbs, 5.85 g Protein, 4.2 g fiber

French Toast with Berries

Preparation time: 10 min

Serves: 2

What you need:

- 2 slice buckwheat bread
- 2 oz. walnut cream
- 2 tbsps. dates syrup
- Blueberries for serving
- 1 tablespoon walnut butter for toping

Method:

1. Mix walnut cream and dates syrup in a bowl.
2. Coat bread slice in cream batter and keep it in the freezer for 10 minutes.
3. Grill bread for 2-3 minutes until slices are cooked and brown.
4. Once cooked remove from grill.
5. Serve with fresh blueberries and walnut butter on top.
6. Serve and enjoy!

Per serving:

Calories Per **Serves:**, 168 kcal, 7.13 g Fat, 25.45 g Total Carbs, 2.44 g Protein, 2.9 g Fiber

Buckwheat Crepe with Berries

Preparation time: 20 min

Serves: 4
What you need:

- 1 cup buckwheat flour
- 2 tbsps. dates syrup
- 1 cup soy milk
- olive oil
- 1 oz. chocolate syrup
- Fresh berries for topping

Method:

1. Mix all crepe ingredients in a bowl.
2. Heat oil in pan over medium heat. Once oil is hot pour ¼ cup buckwheat batter and spread evenly.
3. Cook for 2-3 minutes until golden brown.
4. Flip and cook again for 2-3 minutes.
5. Once cooked remove from heat.
6. Serve with fresh berries and chocolate syrup.
7. Serve and enjoy!

Per serving:

Calories Per **Serves:**, 121 kcal, 0.49 g Fat, 32.2 g Total Carbs, 0.85 g Protein, 5.3 g Fiber

Kiwi & Apple Porridge

Preparation time: 20 min

Serves: 2
What you need:

- 1 cup buckwheat groats
- 2 cups soy milk
- 2 tablespoons date syrup
- 1 tsp cinnamon
- 1 apple chopped
- 1 kiwi, chopped

Topping

- 1 apple, chopped
- 1 kiwi, sliced
- Fresh blueberries

Method:

1. Heat pans over medium heat. Add buckwheat and cook for 10 minutes with milk until cooked through.
2. Add cinnamon, chopped apple, and kiwi.
3. Cook for about 8 minutes, then low the heat and then let it leave for 10 minutes.
4. Top with apple slice, kiwi slice, and fresh berries.
5. Enjoy!

Per serving:
Calories Per **Serves:**, 292 kcal, 10.15 g Fat, 44 g Total Carbs, 10.7 g Protein, 6.2 g Fiber

Strawberry Smoothie Bowl

Preparation time: 5 min

Serves: 1
What you need:

- 1/2 cup walnut milk
- 1 cup strawberries
- 1 tablespoon dates syrup
- Fresh strawberries for topping
- Chia seeds for topping
- Chopped nuts for topping

Method:

1. Blend milk, strawberries, and dates syrup in a blender and blend on high speed.
2. Pour the smoothie in a bowl.
3. Top with strawberries, chia seeds, and berries.
4. Serve cool and enjoy!

Per serving:

Calories Per **Serves:**, 207 kcal, 10.43 g Fat, 27.1 g Total Carbs, 2.42 g Protein, 1.1 g Fiber

Berries Pancakes

Preparation time: 20 min

Serves: 4

What you need:
- 2 apples, puree
- 1 cup, tofu
- 2 teaspoon baking powder
- 2 tbsps. dates syrup
- ¼ teaspoon salt
- 1 tbsp. olive oil
- 1 cup fresh berries for filling
- ¼ cup dates syrup for topping

Method:
1. Mix Pancakes Ingredients in blender and mix well.
2. Pour the mixture into a large bowl and fold in half of the berries
3. Heat your skillet over medium heat and grease it with olive oil
4. Pour pancake batter in skillet and spread it slightly.
5. Cook pancake for 2-3 minutes per side, until cooked through.
6. Serve with fresh berries and dates syrup.
7. Enjoy!

Per serving:
Calories Per **Serves:**, 211 kcal, 4.62 g Fat, 4.43 g Protein, 42.34 g Total Carbs, 6.5 g Fiber

Walnut Cream Parfait

Preparation time: 10 min

Serves: 2
What you need:

- 1 cup walnut cream
- 1 cup cranberries
- 1 tbsp. dates syrup
- Mint leaves
- 1 tbsp. walnuts, chopped

Method:

1. Pour walnut cream in serving glass. Add cranberries then pour cream and dates syrup/
2. Top with dates syrup, mint leaves, and walnuts.
3. Serve cold and enjoy!

Per serving:

Calories Per **Serves:**, 196 kcal, 2.84 g Fat, 12.48 g Protein, 33.05 g

Total Carbs, 1.2 g Fiber

Chocolate Pancakes

Preparation time: 20 min

Serves: 4

What you need:

- 1 cup buckwheat flour
- 2 tbsps. cocoa powder
- 1 tsp baking powder
- 2 tbsp. dates syrup
- 3/4 cup walnut milk
- 1 tsp. olive oil

Method:

1. Mix all pancake ingredients in a mixing bowl until smooth and well incorporated.
2. Heat nonstick griddle over medium heat, and grease with cooking spray.
3. Pour ¼ batter in griddle and Let it cook for 2-3 minutes until cooked.
4. Flip and cook for another 2-3 minutes until cooked through.
5. Stack the pancakes, drizzle chocolate sauce on top, and fresh strawberries.
6. Enjoy!

Per serving:

Calories Per **Serves:**, 169 kcal, 3.57 g Fat, 5.23 g Protein, 31.81 g Total Carbs, 3 g Fiber

Tofu & Spinach Muffins

Preparation time: 30 min

Serves: 12
What you need:

- 1 cup buckwheat flour
- 1 cup tofu, crumbled.
- ¼ cup ground flaxseed
- 2 tsp. baking powder
- ½ tsp salt
- ½ cup walnut milk
- 1 tsp ground cinnamon
- ½ cup dates syrup
- 2 cups spinach, chopped
- ¼ cup walnuts butter

Method:

1. Preheat oven to 375 degrees F.
2. Mix dry ingredients in a bowl and mix well.
3. Mix wet ingredients in a bowl and mix well.
4. Mix wet ingredients to dry mixture and stir to combine.
5. Carefully add chopped spinach to the batter.
6. Pour batter in lined and greased muffin tins.
7. Bake muffins for about 20-25 until cooked through.
8. Serve hot with green juice and enjoy!

Per serving:
Calories Per **Serves:**, 166 kcal, 6.19 g Fat, 3.52 g Protein, 26.94 g
Total Carbs, 3.2 g Fiber

Turmeric Tofu Toast

Preparation time: 10 min

Serves: 4
What you need:

- ½ lb. tofu
- 2 onions, sliced
- 1 tsp. garlic, chopped
- 1 tsp turmeric
- 1/8 tsp. pepper & salt
- 2 tbsps. olive oil
- 4 slice buckwheat bread
- chopped parsley for topping

Method:

1. Heat oil in pan over medium heat, once oil is hot, add garlic and fry.
2. Add onions and fry on low-medium heat for 2-3 minutes.
3. Add crumbled tofu and mash it with a spatula.
4. Season with turmeric, salt, and pepper and mix well.
5. Transfer cooked tofu in plate.
6. Toss bread slice in the same pan.
7. Pour tofu scramble onto warm toast, sprinkle chopped parsley on top.
8. Serve and enjoy!

Per serving:
Calories Per **Serves:**, 263 kcal, 18.6 g Fat, 11.78 g Protein, 16.48 g Total Carbs, 4.1 g Fiber

Apple Bread Loaf

Preparation time: 60 min

Serves: 12

What you need:

- 1/4 cup walnut butter, room temperature
- 2 apples, puree
- 2 tbsps. cocoa powder
- 1/4 cup pure dates sugar
- 2 cups buckwheat flour
- 2 tsps. baking powder

Method:

1. Preheat the oven to 350 degrees F.
2. Grease bread loaf pan with oil and set aside.
3. Mix apple, dates sugar, and butter in a blender and blend.
4. Pour the mixture into a mixing bowl.
5. Add flour, cocoa powder, and baking powder in the bowl and mix well.
6. Pour the batter in greased baking loaf pan.
7. Bake bread for about
8. 40-60 Minutes, or until cooked through.
9. Slice it.
10. Enjoy!

Per serving:

Calories Per **Serves:**, 134 kcal, 4.51 g Fat, 2.65 g Protein, 22.71 g Total Carbs, 2.7 g Fiber

Zucchini Tots

Preparation time: 40 min

Serves: 12

What you need:

- 2 cups buckwheat flour
- ¾ cup soy milk
- 1 tsp. baking powder
- ¼ cup walnut butter
- 1 cup broccoli rice
- 1 zucchini, shredded
- ¼ cup chopped walnuts
- 1 tsp. cinnamon powder

Method:

1. Mix buckwheat flour, walnuts, baking powder, and cinnamon powder in a bowl.
2. Mix milk, butter, zucchini, and broccoli in another bowl,
3. Mix the wet ingredients into the bowl containing the dry ingredients.
4. Preheat the oven to 200 degrees Celsius.
5. Pour batter into each greased muffin cup in the tray.
6. Bake tots for about 20-25 minutes.
7. Once cooked remove from oven.
8. Serve and enjoy!

Per serving:

Calories Per **Serves:**, 122 kcal, 5.89 g Fat, 3.22 g Protein, 15.89 g Total Carbs, 2.4 g Fiber

Tofu & Berries Waffles

Preparation time: 20 min

Serves: 4
What you need:

- 1 cup tofu
- ¼ cup walnut butter
- 1/2 cup walnut milk
- ¼ tsp. cinnamon powder
- 2 tbsps. dates syrup
- 1 tsp. baking powder
- Fresh berries for topping

Method:

1. Turn your waffle maker and set it on medium.
2. Mix all recipe ingredients in blender until smooth and creamy.
3. Pour tofu batter into your waffle maker and cook until the waffle is cooked and crispy.
4. Gently remove the waffles from the machine.
5. Serve with fresh berries on top.
6. Enjoy

Per serving:
Calories Per **Serves:**, 231 kcal, 13.46 g Fat, 4.96 g Protein, 25.45 g

Total Carbs, 3.4 g Fiber

Chocolate Pudding

Preparation time: 30 min

Serves: 6
What you need:

- 8 slice buckwheat bread
- 1 ½ cups walnut milk
- 2 tbsps. dates syrup
- Dark chocolate for topping

Method:

1. Blend bread, walnut milk, and dates syrup in blender.
2. Pour the batter into an oven-safe soufflé dish.
3. Cover and steam pudding for 25 minutes on low to medium flame.
4. Once pudding is cooked, remove it from the dish.
5. Pour melted chocolate on top.
6. Freeze for at least 2 hours.
7. Serve and enjoy!

Per serving:

Calories Per **Serves:**, 239 kcal, 3.17 g Fat, 8.63 g Protein, 48.19 g Total Carbs, 6.1 g Fiber

Cinnamon & Walnut Tea

Preparation time: 5 min

Serves: 2
What you need:

- 2 cups water
- 1 tsp freshly grated ginger root
- 1/2 tsp ground cinnamon
- 1 tbsp. dates syrup
- ¼ cup walnut milk

Method:

1. Heat water in a saucepan over medium heat.
2. Add the ginger, ground cinnamon, dates syrup and cook for about 10 minutes.
3. Pour hot walnut milk, once cooked pour in cup
4. Enjoy!

Per serving:
Calories Per **Serves:**, 38 kcal, 0.09 g Fat, 0.19 g Protein, 10.16 g Total Carbs, 0.7 g Fiber

Apple Porridge

Preparation time: 10 Min

Serves: 4

What you need:

- 2 apples, chopped
- 3 cups walnut milk
- 1 tsp. cinnamon
- 2 tsp. dates syrup
- TOPPING
- Blueberries
- dark chocolate
- apple slice
- walnuts

Method:

1. Mix all ingredients in a bowl that fits inside the bowl of your slow cooker.
2. Place the bowl in your slow cooker, and fill your slow cooker with 1 cup of water to surround the bowl.
3. Cook on LOW 6-8 hours, stirring occasionally.
4. Carefully remove the bowl.
5. Top with banana slices and berries.
6. Serve and enjoy!

Per serving:

Calories Per **Serves:**, 227 kcal, 7.04 g Fat, 36.45 g Total Carbs, 6.95 g Protein, 4.3 g Fiber

Kale Omelet

Preparation time: 20 min

Serves: 2

What you need:
- 2 cups kale, finely chopped
- 1 cup, chopped onion
- 1 cup buckwheat flour
- ¼ cup water
- salt & pepper to taste
- 1 tsp. paprika powder
- 1 tsp. oregano
- olive oil for frying

Method:
1. Mix flour, kale, salt, pepper, oregano, and paprika in a bowl and mix well.
2. Add water slowly in the mixture to make a thick batter.
3. Place a frying pan over medium heat and grease with olive oil.
4. Pour ¼ cup mixture in skillet and spread it evenly.
5. Once cooked, flip and cook for another 2-3 minutes.
6. Once the omelet is cooked remove it from heat.
7. Serve with spinach leaves, tomato slices, and cucumber slices.
8. Enjoy!

Per serving:
Calories Per **Serves:**, 283 kcal, 3.02 g Fat, 57.39 g Total Carbs, 14.52 g Protein, 12.5 g Fiber

Tofu & Kale Toast

Preparation time: 10 min

Serves: 4
What you need:

- 1 tsp. capers, drained and loosely chopped
- sea salt and black pepper
- 1 tsp. sesame seeds
- 1/4 cup guacamole
- 8 oz. tofu, firm and drained
- 4 slices buckwheat bread
- 4 oz. kale
- 1 tbsp. olive oil

Method:

1. Heat olive oil in pan over medium heat and fry tofu until golden brown from all sides.
2. Add capers, salt, and pepper to a mixing bowl.
3. Taste and adjust seasonings as needed.
4. Toast bread on a heated griddle for 2-3 minutes per side.
5. Spread guacamole on each bread slice and arrange on a plate.
6. Arrange tofu on bread slice with kale.
7. Drizzle sesame seeds.
8. Serve and enjoy!

Per serving:
Calories Per **Serves:**, 216 kcal, 17.36 g Fat, 8.43 g Total Carbs, 10.45 g Protein, 3.5 g Fiber

Tofu Scramble

Preparation time: 20 min

Serves: 2
What you need:

- 1 tablespoon olive oil
- 16 oz. block firm tofu
- 1 teaspoon salt
- 1/4 teaspoon turmeric
- 1/4 teaspoon garlic powder
- 2 tablespoons soy milk

Method:

1. Heat the olive oil in a pan over medium heat. Mash the block of tofu right in the pan, with a potato masher or a fork.
2. Cook, stirring frequently, for 3-4 minutes until the water from the tofu is dried.
3. Add salt, turmeric, and garlic powder. Cook and stir constantly for about 5 minutes.
4. Pour the milk into the pan, and stir to mix. Serve immediately.
5. Enjoy!

Per serving:

Calories Per **Serves:**, 208 kcal, 15.44 g Fat, 5.45g Total Carbs, 15.2 g Protein, 0.6 g Fiber

Buckwheat Pancakes

Preparation time: 20 min

Serves: 3
What you need:

- 1 cup buckwheat flour
- 2 tbsps. dates syrup
- 1 cup soya milk
- 1 tbsps. olive oil

Method:

1. Mix all ingredients in a bowl.
2. Heat oil in pan over medium heat. Once oil is hot pour ¼ cup buckwheat batter and spread evenly.
3. Cook for 2-3 minutes until golden brown.
4. Flip and cook again.
5. Once cooked remove from heat.
6. Serve and enjoy!

Per serving:

Calories Per **Serves:**, 197 kcal, 3.92 g Fat, 35.68 g Total Carbs, 7.73 g Protein, 4.43g Fiber

Waffle Sandwich

Preparation time: 10 min

Serves: 4
What you need:

- 1 1/2 cups buckwheat flour
- 2 teaspoons baking powder
- 1 teaspoon baking soda
- 1/4 teaspoon salt
- 1/4 teaspoon cinnamon, optional
- 1 1/2 cups soy milk,
- 1 tablespoon apple cider vinegar
- 1/8 cup olive oil

SERVING

- lettuce leaves
- cucumber slice

Method:

1. Mix all ingredients in a bowl until well incorporated.
2. Preheat a waffle iron and lightly grease with cooking spray. Cook waffles according to the manufacturer's instructions.
3. Serve with lettuce leaves and cucumber slice between two waffles.
4. Enjoy!

Per serving:
Calories Per **Serves:**, 260 kcal, 10.27 g Fat, 38.37 g Total Carbs, 7.16 g Protein, 4.7 g Fiber

Buckwheat Porridge

Preparation time: 10 min

Serves: 4
What you need:

- 1 cup buckwheat groats
- 1 cup chopped kale
- 3 cups water
- 1 tablespoon walnut butter
- ½ tablespoon salt
- ½ cup soya milk
- 1 teaspoon dates syrup

Method:

1. In a saucepan bring water to boil.
2. Add uncooked buckwheat groats. Cover the pot and simmer for 10 minutes (or until water is absorbed).
3. Turn off heat, add the salt, chopped kale, dates syrup and let it sit for 10 more minutes.
4. Top with butter and serve warm in a savory dish, or as a porridge with milk and toppings.

Per serving:

Calories Per **Serves:**, 188 kcal, 4.6 g Fat, 33.56 g Total Carbs, 5.85 g Protein, 4.2 g Fiber

Preparation time: 10 min

Serves: 2

What you need:

- 2 slice buckwheat bread slices2 oz. chocolate cream
- 1 cup apple
- 2 tbsps. dates syrup
- 1/2 cup water

Method:

1. Grill bread for 2 minutes.
2. Heat water in a pan over medium heat.
3. Add dates syrup and apple and cook for 5-8 minutes until apples are soft and caramelize.
4. Spread chocolate cream over the grill bread slice.
5. Sprinkle caramelize apple on top.
6. Serve and enjoy!

Per serving:

Calories Per **Serves:**, 168 kcal, 7.13 g Fat, 25.45 g Total Carbs, 2.44 g Protein, 2.9 g Fiber

MAIN MEALS

Creamy Spinach Curry

Preparation time: 20 Min

Serves: 4

What you need:

- 1 lb. spinach, chopped
- 1 tsp. ginger garlic paste
- salt & pepper to taste
- 1 tsp. paprika powder
- 1 tsp. cumin seeds
- 1 tsp red chili powder
- 1/2 tsp. turmeric powder
- 1 tbsp. olive oil
- ½ cup walnut cream

Method:

1. Heat the oil in a pan over medium heat.
2. Once the oil is hot, add ginger garlic paste and cook for a minute.
3. Add chopped spinach in pan and cook for 4-5 minutes until spinach is welted.
4. Add rest of the spices and mix well.
5. Blender spinach in blender for 1 minute.
6. Pour spinach in a pan again, add walnut cream and cook on low heat for about 4-5 minutes.
7. Once cooked remove from heat, drizzle cream on top.
8. Enjoy!

Per serving:

Calories Per **Serves:**, 125 kcal, 9.84 g Fat, 4.51 g Protein, 7.47 g Total Carbs, 3.1 g Fiber

Broccoli Olives Pizza

Preparation time: 30 min

Serves: 8
What you need:

- 1 lb. buckwheat pizza dough
- 2 tbsp. olive oil
- 1 bunch broccoli, cut into florets.
- 1 red onion, sliced
- 1 tsp minced garlic
- salt & pepper to taste
- 1 oz. BBQ sauce
- 2 oz. olives
- 6 oz. tofu, sliced

Method:

1. Heat oil in skillet over medium heat.
2. Once the oil is hot, sauté onion and garlic for 2-3 minutes.
3. Season with spices and mix well.
4. Add broccoli in skillet and cook for about 5 minutes.
5. Preheat oven to 400.
6. Set buckwheat pizza dough over greased pizza pan.
7. Cover dough with BBQ sauce. Layer with tofu sliced, cooked broccoli, and broccoli.
8. Bake for about 10 minutes.
9. Serve hot and enjoy!

Per serving:

Calories Per **Serves:**, 296 kcal, 10.7 g Fat, 11.44 g Protein, 44.03 g Total Carbs, 6.9 g Fiber

Buffalo Broccoli Bites

Preparation time: 40 min

Serves: 4
What you need:

- 1 head of broccoli, cut into bite-sized florets
- 1 cup buckwheat flour
- 3/4 cup soy milk
- 2 tsps. garlic powder
- 1 1/2 tsps. paprika powder
- salt &black pepper
- 1 tsp. oregano
- 3/4 cup breadcrumbs
- 1 cup spicy BBQ sauce

Method:

1. Mix flour, soy milk, water, garlic powder, paprika powder, salt, and black pepper in a mixing bowl.
2. Dip the florets into the batter until they are coated well.
3. Roll florets over the breadcrumbs.
4. Arrange the florets over a baking tray and bake for 25 minutes at 350 °F.
5. Transfer the cooked broccoli bits to a bowl and coat BBQ sauce over it and bake again for 20 minutes at 350 °F.
6. Serve immediately and enjoy!

Per serving:

Calories Per **Serves:**, 161 kcal, 2.77 g Fat, 7.62 g Protein, 30.1 g Total Carbs, 5.5 g Fiber

Spinach Soup

Preparation time: 20 Min

Serves: 4

What you need:

- 1 lb. spinach, chopped
- 1 tsp. ginger garlic paste
- salt & pepper to taste
- 1 tsp. paprika powder
- 1 tsp. cumin seeds
- 1 tsp red chili powder
- 1/2 tsp. turmeric powder
- 1 tbsp. olive oil
- 3 cups vegetable broth

Method:

1. Heat the oil in a pan over medium heat.
2. Once the oil is hot, add ginger garlic paste and cook for a minute.
3. Add chopped spinach in pan and cook for 4-5 minutes until spinach is welted.
4. Add rest of the spices and mix well.
5. Blender spinach in blender for 1 minute.
6. Pour spinach in a pan again, add broth and cook on low heat for about 4-5 minutes.
7. Once cooked remove from heat, drizzle cream on top.
8. Enjoy

Per serving:

Calories Per **Serves:**, 67 kcal, 4.05 g Fat, 3.7 g Protein, 6.37 g Total Carbs, 3.1 g Fiber

Chili Tofu

Preparation time: 20 Min

Serves: 4

What you need:

- 8 oz. tofu cut into cubes
- 1 tbsp. extra-virgin olive oil
- 2 large garlic cloves, minced
- 1 tsp. chili flakes
- salt & pepper
- 1 red chili, cut into rings
- 2 tbsps. green onion
- Salt and freshly ground black pepper

Method:

1. Heat a large heavy skillet over medium heat. Add the oil, once the oil is hot, add the tofu with garlic cook for 5-8 minutes until brown.
2. Season with spices and add red chili rings.
3. Drizzle green onion on top.
4. Serve and enjoy!

Per serving:

Calories Per **Serves:**, 174 kcal, 12.99 g Fat, 10.02 g Protein, 7.56 g Total Carbs, 2.5 g Fiber

Spicy Spinach Fillet

Preparation time: 20 min

Serves: 4
What you need:

- 1 cup buckwheat Flour
- 2 cups spinach, chopped
- 1/2 cup Onions, chopped
- 1 tsp. red chill
- 1/2 cup Kale, chopped
- 2 tsp. Basil
- 2 tsp. Oregano
- ½ cup water
- Olive Oil for frying

Method:

1. Mix all seasonings and vegetables in a large bowl.
2. Add flour and spicy in the same bowl with seasoning and mix.
3. Add water to this mixture and mix.
4. The mixture should be thick enough to make patties.
5. Heat oil in skillet over medium heat.
6. Once the oil is hot, cook patties in skillet for about 2-3 minutes.
7. Flip and cook for another 2-3 minutes until both sides are brown.
8. Serve with tomato slices and enjoy.

Per serving:

Calories Per **Serves:**, 119 kcal, 1.07 g Fat, 4.75 g Protein, 25.11 g Total Carbs, 4.1 g Fiber

Broccoli Patties

Preparation time: 20 min

Serves: 4

What you need:

- 1 cup buckwheat Flour
- 1 cup broccoli, chopped
- 1/2 cup Onions, chopped
- 1/2 cup Green Peppers, chopped
- 1/2 cup Kale, chopped
- 2 tsp. Basil
- 2 tsp. Oregano
- 2 tsp. Onion Powder
- 1/2 tsp. Ginger Powder
- ½ cup water
- Olive Oil for frying

Method:

1. Mix all seasonings and vegetables in a large bowl.
2. Add flour and broccoli in the same bowl with seasoning and mix thoroughly.
3. Add water to this mixture and mix.
4. The mixture should be thick enough to make patties.
5. Heat oil in skillet over medium heat.
6. Once the oil is hot, cook patties in skillet for about 2-3 minutes.
7. Flip and cook for another 2-3 minutes until both sides are brown.
8. Serve hot and enjoy!

Per serving:

Calories Per **Serves:**, 117 kcal, 1.06 g Fat, 4.63 g Protein, 24.85 g Total Carbs, 4.1 g Fiber

Spinach & Tofu Pizza

Preparation time: 40 Min

Serves: 8

What you need:

- 1/2 lb. spinach, trimmed
- 1 lb. buckwheat pizza dough.
- 16 oz. tofu, cut into cubes
- salt & pepper to taste
- 1 tsp oregano
- 1 tsp. chili powder
- 1 tbsp. olive oil
- 1 oz. walnut cream

Method:

1. Preheat the oven to 400°F.
2. Sautee spinach in a skillet over medium heat, for about 10 minutes until spinach is wilted.
3. Season with spices and mix well.
4. Set pizza dough over greased pizza pan.
5. Spread the walnut cream over pizza dough then spread spinach.
6. Top with tofu bites.
7. Bake pizza for about 20 minutes in preheated oven.
8. Once cooked remove from oven.
9. Serve and enjoy.

Per serving:

Calories Per **Serves:**, 254 kcal, 15.93 g Fat, 13.17 g Protein, 19.63 g Total Carbs, 4.8 g Fiber

Broccoli Flatbread Pizza

Preparation time: 30 min

Serves: 8
What you need:

- 1 lb. buckwheat dough
- 2 tbsp. olive oil
- 1 bunch broccoli, cut into florets.
- 1 red onion, sliced
- 1 tsp minced garlic
- salt & pepper to taste
- 1 oz. walnut cream

Method:

1. Heat oil in skillet over medium heat.
2. Once the oil is hot, sauté onion and garlic for 2-3 minutes.
3. Season with spices and mix well.
4. Add broccoli in skillet and cook for about 5 minutes.
5. Preheat oven to 400.
6. Set buckwheat dough over greased pizza pan.
7. Cover dough with walnut cream. Layer with cooked broccoli.
8. Bake for about 10 minutes.
9. Serve hot and enjoy!

Per serving:

Calories Per **Serves:**, 112 kcal, 6.13 g Fat, 3.08 g Protein, 12.97 g Total Carbs, 2.3 g Fiber

Turmeric Spinach Patties

Preparation time: 20 min

Serves: 4

What you need:

- 1 cup buckwheat Flour
- 2 cups spinach, chopped
- 1/2 cup Onions, chopped
- 1 tbsp. turmeric
- 1/2 cup Kale, chopped
- 2 tsp. Basil
- 2 tsp. Oregano
- 2 tsp. Onion Powder
- 1/2 tsp. Ginger Powder
- ½ cup spring water
- Olive oil for frying

Method:

1. Mix all seasonings and vegetables in a large bowl.
2. Add flour and spinach in the same bowl with seasoning and mix thoroughly.
3. Add water to this mixture and mix.
4. The mixture should be thick enough to make patties.
5. Heat oil in skillet over medium heat.
6. Once the oil is hot, cook patties in skillet for about 2-3 minutes._Flip and cook for another 2-3 minutes until both sides are brown.
7. Serve hot and enjoy!

Per serving:

Calories Per **Serves:**, 124 kcal, 1.13 g Fat, 4.86 g Protein, 26.16 g Total Carbs, 4.6 g Fiber

Stir Fried Broccoli & Tofu

Preparation time: 20 Min

Serves: 4

What you need:

- 8 oz. tofu cut into cubes
- 16 oz. broccoli cut into
- 1 tbsp. extra-virgin olive oil
- 2 large garlic cloves, minced
- Salt and freshly ground black pepper
- 2 oz. walnut cream
- Spinach leaves

Method:

1. Heat a large heavy skillet over medium heat. Add the oil, once the oil is hot, add broccoli with garlic and cook for 4-8 minutes until cooked.
2. Transfer cooked broccoli to a plate.
3. Add the tofu cook for another 5-8 minutes until brown.
4. Transfer cooked tofu with broccoli and assemble spinach with them.
5. Drizzle walnut cream, salt, and pepper on top.
6. Serve and enjoy!

Per serving:

Calories Per **Serves:**, 287 kcal, 22.75 g Fat, 15.81 g Protein, 11.62 g Total Carbs, 6.3 g Fiber

Wilted Spinach with Onion

Preparation time: 40 Min

Serves: 2

What you need:

- 4 red onions, cut into rings
- 1/4 cup olive oil
- 2 1lb. spinach with stems
- Salt and freshly ground pepper

Method:

1. Heat oil in a large pan over medium heat.
2. Add the onion rings and cook for about 10-15 minutes over low heat until the onion is caramelized.
3. Transfer onion to plate.
4. Add spinach in the same pan and cook for about 5-10 minutes until about to wilted.
5. Transfer spinach to plate.
6. Top with caramelized onion.
7. Drizzle salt & pepper on top.
8. Serve and enjoy!

Per serving:

Calories Per **Serves:**, 300 kcal, 22.79 g Fat, 13.6 g Protein, 18.13 g Total Carbs, 11.1 g Fiber

Broccoli with Garlic sauce

Preparation time: 30 Min

Serves: 2

What you need:
- 1/3 cup minced fresh garlic
- 2 tablespoons olive oil
- 1 head broccoli cut into florets with stems
- 1 cup vegetable broth
- 1 tsp. turmeric
- salt & pepper to taste
- 1 tbsp. buckwheat flour

Method:
1. Heat oil in skillet over medium he
2. Add broccoli florets and cook for 4-5 minutes. Set aside.
3. Add minced garlic in the same skillet and cook for 3 - 5 minutes, until garlic begins to brown.
4. Add broth salt & pepper and flour and mix well.
5. Pour broccoli in skillet again and cook for another 4-5 minutes until broccoli is soft and sauce is thick.
6. Serve hot and enjoy!

Per serving:
Calories Per **Serves:**, 282 kcal, 14.95 g Fat, 11.07 g Protein, 33.39 g Total Carbs, 9.4 g Fiber

Hot & Sour Spinach

Preparation time: 40 Min

Serves: 2

What you need:
- 1 red onion, minced
- 1/2 cup sherry vinegar
- 1 thyme sprig
- 1 tablespoon dates syrup
- 2 1lb. spinach
- 3 tablespoons extra-virgin olive oil
- Salt and freshly ground pepper
- 1 cup vegetable broth

Method:
1. Heat oil in pan over medium heat.
2. Add the onion and cook for about 2-3 minutes over low heat.
3. Add the vinegar and thyme sprig and bring to a boil.
4. Simmer over low heat until the vinegar is reduced.
5. Add dates syrup and mix well.
6. Add broth in pan, bring to a boil.
7. Add the spinach and cook until wilted.
8. Season with salt and pepper and cook for about 5 minutes.
9. Transfer the spinach to a platter with some broth.
10. Serve and enjoy!

Per serving:
Calories Per **Serves:**, 296 kcal, 11.86 g Fat, 15.79 g Protein, 37.91 g Total Carbs, 12.3 g Fiber

Spinach & Tofu Curry

Preparation time: 30 Min

Serves: 4
What you need:
- 2 cups, tofu cubes
- 2 cups spinach, chopped
- 2 cloves
- 1 cardamom
- 2 tbsps. olive oil
- 1 green chili, chopped
- 1 onion, chopped
- 1 cup walnut milk
- ½ tsp. ginger-garlic paste
- 1 tsp. cumin seeds
- Salt to taste

Method:
1. Heat oil in a pan over medium heat. once oil is hot, add tofu cubes and cook for 2-3 minutes.
2. Transfer fried tofu in plate.
3. Add the clove, cardamom, cinnamon, and cumin seeds and onion in pan and cook for 2-3 minutes.
4. Add spinach, milk, salt, and ginger-garlic paste.
5. Stir-fry for 10-15 minutes over medium heat
6. Add fried tofu stir and combine well.
7. Once cooked remove from heat.
8. Serve and enjoy!

Per serving:
Calories Per **Serves:**, 237 kcal, 11.31 g Fat, 7.34 g Protein, 27.12 g Total Carbs, 1.1 g Fiber

Sardine Puttanesca Spaghetti

Preparation time: 10 Min

Serves: 4

What you need:
- 300-400 g buckwheat spaghetti
- 1 tbsp olive
- 2 garlic cloves, minced
- 1/4 tsp chill flakes, optional
- 2 tin chopped tomatoes
- 1 tin sardines in olive oil
- 2 tbsp pitted black olives, sliced
- 1 tbsp capers
- 2 cups frozen chopped kale
- handful of fresh parsley or chives, roughly chopped

Method:
1. Bring a large pan of water to the boil and add a generous pinch of salt. When the water is boiling, add the spaghetti and simmer for 8-10 mins until al dente while you make the sauce.
2. Heat the oil in a large frying pan and add the garlic and chili flakes.
3. Cook for 30 secs-1 min then add the chopped tomatoes.
4. Cook for a couple of mins, then add the sardines, olives, capers, and kale.
5. Cook for another 4-5 mins, until sauce is cooked, sardines are broken up in the sauce and everything is heated through.
6. Drain the spaghetti and stir the sauce through it, then serve with the fresh herbs.

Per serving:
Calories Per **Serves:**, 237 kcal, 11.31 g Fat, 7.34 g Protein, 27.12 g Total Carbs, 1.1 g Fiber

Tofu Power Bowls

Preparation time: 50 Min

Serves: 4

What you need:
- 1 cup buckwheat groats
- 1 package extra-firm tofu
- 1/2 tablespoons cornstarch
- 1 1/2 teaspoons chili powder
- 1 teaspoon kosher salt
- 1/2 teaspoon freshly ground black pepper
- 1/2 teaspoon garlic powder
- 2 teaspoons olive oil
- 2 cups shredded kale
- 1 1/2 cups shelled cooked edamame
- 2 carrots, peeled and grated
- 3/4 cup packed fresh cilantro leaves
- 1 lime, cut into wedges

For the creamy walnut sauce
- 1/4 cup creamy walnut butter
- 1 tablespoon reduced sodium soy sauce
- 1 tablespoon freshly squeezed lime juice
- 2 teaspoons dark brown sugar
- 1 teaspoon sambal oelek
- 1 teaspoon freshly grated ginger

Method:
1. To make the walnut sauce, mix walnut butter, soy sauce, lime juice, brown sugar, sambal oelek, ginger, and 2-3 tablespoons water in a small bowl and set aside.
2. Cook buckwheat in water and cook for few minutes.
3. Preheat oven to 400 degrees F. Line a baking sheet with parchment paper.

4. In a large bowl mix crumbled tofu, cornstarch, chili powder, salt, pepper, and garlic powder. Stir in 1 tablespoon olive oil until well combined.
5. Bake tofu for 30 minutes, until golden brown and crispy.
6. In a small bowl, add kale and drizzle with the remaining 2 teaspoons olive oil; season with salt and pepper to taste. Massage until the kale starts to soften and wilt, about 1-2 minutes.
7. Divide buckwheat into bowls.
8. Top with tofu, kale, edamame, carrots, and cilantro.
9. Serve with creamy walnut sauce.
10. Enjoy!

Per serving:
Calories Per **Serves:**, 237 kcal, 11.31 g Fat, 7.34 g Protein, 27.12 g Total Carbs, 1.1 g Fiber

Superfood Bibimbap With Crispy Tofu

Preparation time: 45 Min

Serves: 4

What you need:

- 1 block organic extra firm tofu, sliced
- 1/2 cup low sodium soy sauce
- 1-2 tablespoons chili paste
- tablespoons toasted sesame oil
- 1-inch fresh ginger, grated
- cloves garlic, grated
- 2 tablespoons extra virgin olive oil
- cup shiitake mushrooms, sliced or torn
- 1 bunch curly kale, roughly torn
- juice from 1 lime
- kosher salt
- 2 cups cooked buckwheat
- 1 avocado, sliced
- 1 cup fresh or pickled carrots and radishes

Method:

1. Preheat the oven to 400 degrees F. Line a baking sheet with parchment paper.
2. Slice into 1/4-inch-thick slices and add to a gallon size Ziplock bag.
3. In a small bowl, mix the 2-tablespoon water, the soy sauce, chili paste, sesame oil, ginger, and garlic. Add half the sauce to the tofu bag tossing gently to combine. Let it sit for 5-10 minutes.
4. Remove the tofu from the sauce and bake for 10 minutes. Flip and bake another 10-15 minutes, until the tofu is crisp.
5. Meanwhile, toss mushrooms with 1 tablespoon oil and a pinch of salt.
6. Add the veggies to the pan with the tofu.

7. In a bowl, massage the kale with the remaining 1 tablespoons olive oil, lime juice, and a pinch of salt.
8. Divide the grains among bowls. Add the tofu, kale, mushrooms, avocado, carrots, and radishes.
9. Enjoy!

Per serving:

Calories Per **Serves:**, 237 kcal, 11.31 g Fat, 7.34 g Protein, 27.12 g Total Carbs, 1.1 g Fiber

Spicy Tofu Kale Wraps

Preparation time: 20 Min

Serves: 2

What you need:

- 3 tablespoons soy sauce
- 2 tablespoon sesame oil
- 1-3 teaspoons chili paste
- 2 teaspoons ginger
- 2 teaspoons sugar
- 2 teaspoon rice vinegar
- 2 cloves garlic, minced
- 2 tablespoon vegetable oil
- 1 (12-ounce) package firm tofu
- 1 red bell pepper, diced
- 2 cups chopped mushrooms
- Kale leaves, for serving

Method:

1. In a small bowl, mix soy sauce, sesame oil, chili paste, ginger, sugar, rice vinegar, and garlic; set aside.
2. Heat vegetable oil in a skillet over medium heat.
3. Add tofu and sear until golden brown, about 2-3 minutes on each side. Transfer to a paper towel-lined plate.
4. Add mushrooms and bell pepper to skillet and cook, stirring frequently until tender, about 3-4 minutes.
5. Stir in soy sauce mixture and cook until sauce has reduced slightly, about 2-3 minutes.
6. To serve, spoon several tablespoons of the tofu mixture into the center of a kale leaf.
7. Serve and enjoy!

Per serving:

Calories Per **Serves:**, 237 kcal, 11.31 g Fat, 7.34 g Protein, 27.12 g Total Carbs, 1.1 g Fiber

Tofu Burritos

Preparation time: 35 Min

Serves: 8

What you need:
- 8 Tortillas

For eggless egg salad
- 12 oz tofu extra firm
- 1/3 cup vegenaise
- tbsp yellow mustard
- 1/4 tsp cayenne pepper
- 1 tsp turmeric
- tbsp fresh parsley chopped
- 1 tbsp dill chopped
- tbsp fresh cilantro chopped
- green onions chopped
- 1 cup cherry tomatoes chopped
- 1 tbsp lime juice
- salt and pepper to taste
- 1/2 tsp salt or to taste
- 1/4 tsp pepper or to taste

Method:
1. In a large bowl crumble up the tofu using your hands.
2. Add the remaining ingredients for the eggless egg salad and stir well.
3. Adjust seasoning with salt and pepper as necessary.
4. To assemble the burritos, top each tortilla with 1/2 cup of the eggless egg salad.
5. Roll up the burritos and wrap them in foil.
6. Refrigerate leftover burritos wrapped in foil for about 2 to 3 days.
7. You can also heat them a bit in the microwave before serving.

Per serving:
Calories Per **Serves:**, 237 kcal, 11.31 g Fat, 7.34 g Protein, 27.12 g Total Carbs, 1.1 g Fiber

Asian Garlic Tofu

Preparation time: 60 Min

Serves: 2

What you need:

- 1 package super firm tofu
- 1/4 cup Hoisin sauce
- 2 tablespoons soy sauce
- 1 teaspoon sugar
- 1 teaspoon freshly grated ginger
- 2 cloves garlic, minced
- 1/4 teaspoon red pepper flakes
- 1 tablespoon olive oil
- 1 teaspoon sesame oil
- green onions for garnish
- rice for serving

Method:

1. Remove tofu from packaging. Place about 4 paper towels on a plate. Set tofu on top of the plate and cover with more paper towels. Place a cast iron pan or something else that is heavy on top. Let it sit for 30 minutes.
2. In a medium bowl, stir together Hoisin sauce, soy sauce, sugar, ginger, garlic, and red pepper flakes.
3. Cut tofu into bite-sized pieces. Place in bowl with sauce and toss to coat. Let sit for 30 minutes.
4. Heat olive oil in a medium cast-iron pan over medium-high heat. Once really hot, add tofu. Once nicely seared on the bottom, flip over. Continue to cook until seared on the bottom.
5. Drizzle with sesame oil and remove from heat.
6. Sprinkle with green onions.
7. Enjoy!

Per serving:

Calories Per **Serves:**, 237 kcal, 11.31 g Fat, 7.34 g Protein, 27.12 g Total Carbs, 1.1 g Fiber

Tofu Burritos Recipe 2

Preparation time: 35 Min

Serves: 8

What you need:

- 16 oz soft tofu cut into 1/2-inch cubes
- ¼ lb. ground pork
- 1/2 tbsp sesame oil
- o 1/2 tbsp doubanjiang roughly chopped
- 1 tbsp chili oil
- 1 cup water
- 1 tbsp low sodium soy sauce
- 2 garlic cloves minced
- 1 tsp grated ginger
- 1 tsp sugar
- 1-1/2 tbsp water + 1 tbsp cornstarch
- 2 green scallions, finely sliced
- 1/2 tsp Sichuan peppercorn powder

Method:

1. To make peppercorn powder, fry 1 heaping tbsp of peppercorns in a small skillet with about 1 tsp of oil (any kind). Toss peppercorn until the aroma of peppercorns comes out. Pat dry and let cool. Place in a spice grinder and grind to powder. Set aside.
2. Bring a large pot of water to boil. Slide in tofu. Cook for about 1 minute. Drain tofu and set aside.
3. In a large skillet, add the ground pork and sesame oil and cook until pork is cooked. Then add in the doubanjiang, garlic, ginger, chili oil. Cook for about 1 minute.
4. Add in 1 cup of water. Bring to a boil and slide in tofu. Stir in soy sauce and sugar. Taste and adjust seasoning as needed. You can add more soy sauce if you feel it isn't salty enough. If you feel it isn't spicy enough you

can add more chili oil or more doubanjiang. Keep in mind that you will also be adding peppercorn powder at the end which will add to the spiciness. If it is too spicy, you can add a little more sugar. Cook until sauce is reduced.

5. In a small bowl add 2 1/2 tbsp water and 1 tbsp cornstarch. Stir until cornstarch is completely dissolved into water. Add to sauce and immediately stir so that the cornstarch slurry dissolves into the sauce and doesn't clump up. Cook about 30 more seconds or until sauce is thickened.

6. Turn off heat and sprinkle peppercorn powder and scallions over the dish. If desired, you can also drizzle with a little more chili oil.

7. Serve immediately with rice or rice substitute of your choice.

Per serving:

Calories Per **Serves:**, 237 kcal, 11.31 g Fat, 7.34 g Protein, 27.12 g Total Carbs, 1.1 g Fiber

Hot & Sour Soup

Preparation time: 20 Min

Serves: 4

What you need:

- 6 cups chicken or vegetable broth
- 14-ounce package water-packed extra-firm tofu, drained
- 1 cup mushrooms, thinly sliced
- 1/2 cup bamboo shoots
- 1/3 cup rice wine vinegar
- 6 tablespoons low sodium soy sauce
- 2 teaspoons minced garlic
- 2teaspoon Gourmet Ginger
- 1/2 teaspoon crushed red pepper flakes

Method:

1. Chop tofu into cubes and set aside.
2. Mix broth, vinegar, soy sauce, garlic, ginger, and crushed red pepper flakes in a large pot and bring to a boil.
3. Add in tofu, mushrooms, and bamboo shoots and cook on heat to medium-low.
4. Cook 5-10 minutes longer.
5. Garnish with dried cilantro or chives and serve immediately.

Per serving:

Calories Per **Serves:**, 237 kcal, 11.31 g Fat, 7.34 g Protein, 27.12 g Total Carbs, 1.1 g Fiber

Tofu & Avocado Spring Rolls

Preparation time: 20 Min

Serves: 4

What you need:

Walnut dipping sauce

- 1/2 cup creamy walnut butter
- 2/3 cup water
- 2 Tablespoons hoisin sauce
- splash of fish sauce (optional)
- 2 garlic cloves, minced
- 1 teaspoon sugar

Buckwheat noodles, cooked according to instructions on the package

- 1 pound firm tofu, sliced and then cut into strips
- 1 tbsp. olive oil
- 1/2 red pepper, sliced into strips
- 1 avocado, sliced
- 1/2 cucumber, cut into strips
- 1/4 purple cabbage, sliced
- Thai basil leaves
- rice paper rice paper

Method:

1. Mix walnut sauce Ingredients in a small mixing bowl.
2. Cook the noodles according to the instructions on the bag or box of noodles. After cutting the tofu into strips, place on a dry, clean paper towel.
3. Heat the oil on medium to medium-high for 4 to 5 minutes. Cook the tofu for about 4 to 5 minutes on each side.
4. Place on a plate lined with clean paper towels.
5. One at a time, wet the rice paper and then place it on a round plate.

6. Allow the rice paper to sit for at least one minute.
7. Add noodles, tofu, red pepper, avocado, cucumber, cabbage, and a couple of basil leaves and roll it.
8. Serve with the walnut dipping sauce.

Per serving:

Calories Per **Serves:**, 237 kcal, 11.31 g Fat, 7.34 g Protein, 27.12 g Total Carbs, 1.1 g Fiber

Simple Tofu Quiche

Preparation time: 45 Min

Serves: 8

What you need:

Crust

- 3 medium-large potatoes, grated and squeezed
- 2 Tbsp melted vegan butter
- 1/4 tsp sea salt and pepper

Filling

- 12.3 ounces extra-firm silken tofu
- 2 Tbsp nutritional yeast
- 3 Tbsp hummus
- Sea salt and black pepper (to taste)
- 3 cloves garlic (chopped)
- 2 medium leeks chopped
- 3/4 cup cherry tomatoes (halved)
- 1 cup chopped kale

Method:

1. Preheat oven to 450 degrees F (232 C) and grease quiche pan with cooking spray.
2. Add potatoes to a pie dish and drizzle with melted vegan butter and 1/4 tsp each salt and pepper. Toss to coat, then use fingers to press into the pan and up the sides to form an even layer.
3. Bake for 25-30 minutes or until golden brown all over. Set aside.
4. Prep veggies and garlic and add to a baking sheet. Toss with 2 Tbsp olive oil and a healthy pinch of each salt and pepper and toss to coat.
5. Place in the oven and bake until soft and golden brown (a total of 20-30 minutes). Set aside and lower oven heat to 375 degrees F (190 C).

6. Add drained tofu to a food processor with nutritional yeast, hummus, and a heaping 1/4 tsp each sea salt and black pepper. Set aside.
7. Remove veggies from the oven, add to a mixing bowl, and top with the tofu mixture. Toss to coat, then add to the crust and spread into an even layer.
8. Bake quiche at 375 degrees F (190 C) for a total of 30–40 minutes
9. Serve and enjoy!

Per serving:
Calories Per **Serves:**, 237 kcal, 11.31 g Fat, 7.34 g Protein, 27.12 g Total Carbs, 1.1 g Fiber

Barbecued Waffle Iron Tofu

Preparation time: 10 Min

Serves: 2

What you need:
- 7 - 8 ounces extra-firm tofu
- 3 tablespoons Ketchup or tomato sauce
- 1 teaspoon barbecue seasoning
- 1/2 teaspoon soy sauce or gluten-free tamari
- 1/4 teaspoon spicy brown mustard or other prepared mustard
- 1 pinch stevia

Method:
1. Drain the tofu and cut it into 3-4 equally thick pieces lengthwise.
2. On a shallow plate, mix the ketchup or tomato sauce with the barbecue rub, soy sauce, and mustard.
3. Combine well and add stevia. Drag each piece of tofu through the sauce until it's coated on all sides.
4. Preheat your waffle iron on its highest setting. Once it is hot, place the tofu on the iron, distributing it equally. Gently close the waffle iron and set a timer for 4-5 minutes.
5. Brush waffles with extra barbecue sauce and serve alone or on sandwiches.

Per serving:
Calories Per **Serves:**, 237 kcal, 11.31 g Fat, 7.34 g Protein, 27.12 g Total Carbs, 1.1 g Fiber

Cauliflower Mac 'n' Cheese

Preparation time: 30 Min

Serves: 8

What you need:

- 3 tbsp. olive oil, divided, plus more for baking dish
- lb. buckwheat pasta
- medium-sized head cauliflower, florets
- 4 cloves garlic, sliced
- large yellow onion, thinly sliced
- Kosher salt and freshly ground black pepper
- 8 oz. tofu crumbled
- 1/4 tsp. mustard powder
- Pinch cayenne pepper
- 1/2 cup panko breadcrumbs
- 1/2 cup kale leaves chopped

Method:

1. Cook pasta according to package **Method:**.
2. Heat 2 tablespoons oil in a large pot over medium heat. Add cauliflower, garlic, and onion. Season with salt. Cook, covered, stirring occasionally, until tender, 15 to 20 minutes. Add 4 cups water and simmer until vegetables are very soft, 10 to 12 minutes. Drain, reserving 2 cups cooking liquid; let cool slightly.
3. Mix vegetables, tofu, mustard powder, and cayenne in a blender.
4. Purée, adding just enough reserved cooking liquid to get the mixture moving, until smooth, 1 to 2 minutes.
5. Add sauce to pasta and toss to combine. Transfer to prepared baking dish. Toss together panko, kale, and the remaining tablespoon of oil in a bowl.
6. Season with salt and pepper. Sprinkle over pasta.
7. Serve and enjoy!

Per serving:

Calories Per **Serves:**, 237 kcal, 11.31 g Fat, 7.34 g Protein, 27.12 g Total Carbs, 1.1 g Fiber

Beans & Broccolini

Preparation time: 15 Min

Serves: 4

What you need:

- Kosher salt and freshly ground black pepper
- 1 lb. Broccolini, trimmed
- tbsp. olive oil
- tsp. lemon zest, plus 2 tablespoons juice
- tbsp. capers, drained and chopped
- tbsp. honey mustard
- 1/2 red pepper flakes
- 1 (15.5-ounce) can small white beans, rinsed

Method:

1. Boil Broccolini in salted water and cook until stalks are crisp-tender, 1 to 2 minutes.
2. Whisk together oil, lemon zest and juice, capers, mustard, and red pepper flakes in a bowl.
3. Season with salt and pepper.
4. Add Broccolini and beans; toss to coat.

Per serving:

Calories Per **Serves:**, 237 kcal, 11.31 g Fat, 7.34 g Protein, 27.12 g Total Carbs, 1.1 g Fiber

Chicken Stew

Preparation time: 20 Min

Serves: 4

What you need:
- **2** tablespoons extra-virgin olive oil
- **1** yellow onion, chopped
- **1** tablespoon garlic, minced
- **1** tablespoon fresh ginger, minced
- **1** teaspoon ground turmeric
- **1** teaspoon ground cumin
- **1** teaspoon ground coriander
- **1** teaspoon paprika
- 4 (6-ounce) boneless, skinless chicken thighs, trimmed and cut into **1**-inch pieces
- 4 tomatoes, chopped
- **14** oz. walnut milk
- Salt and ground black pepper, as required
- 6 cups fresh Swiss chard, chopped
- **2** tablespoons fresh lemon juice

Method:
1. Heat olive oil in a large heavy-bottomed soup pan over medium heat and sauté the onion for about 3- 4 minutes.
2. Add the ginger, garlic, and spices, and sauté for about **1** minute.
3. Add the chicken and cook for about 4-5 minutes.
4. Add the tomatoes, coconut milk, salt, and black pepper, and bring to a gentle simmer.
5. Adjust the heat to low and simmer, covered for about **10-1**5 minutes.
6. Stir in the Swiss chard and cook for about 4-5 minutes.
7. Add in lemon juice and remove from the heat.
8. Serve hot.

Baked Chicken with Salad

Preparation time: 40 Min

Serves: 4

What you need:

For Chicken

- 4 boneless, skinless chicken breast halves
- Salt and ground black pepper, as required
- 2 tablespoons extra-virgin olive oil

For Salad

- 4 cups fresh kale, tough ribs removed and chopped
- 2 cups carrots, peeled and julienned
- ¼ cup walnuts

For Dressing

- 1 small garlic clove, minced
- 2 tablespoons fresh lime juice
- 2 tablespoons extra-virgin olive oil
- 1 teaspoon raw honey
- ½ teaspoon Dijon mustard
- Salt and ground black pepper, as required

Method:

1. Season chicken breast half with salt and black pepper evenly.
2. Heat the oil in a **12**-inch sauté pan over medium-low heat.
3. Place the chicken breast and cook for about 9-**10** minutes, without moving.
4. Flip the chicken breasts and cook for about 6 minutes or until cooked through.
5. Remove the sauté pan from heat and let the chicken stand in the pan for about 3 minutes.
9. Transfer the chicken breasts onto a cutting board for about 5 minutes.

10. Place all ingredients in a salad bowl and mix.
11. Mix all ingredients in another bowl and beat until well combined.
12. Cut each chicken breast into desired-sized slices.
13. Place the salad onto each serving plate and top each with chicken slices.
14. Drizzle with dressing and serve.

Lamb Chops with Salad

Preparation time: 40 Min

Serves: 4

What you need:

For Lamb Chops

- **2** tablespoons extra-virgin olive oil, divided
- 4 garlic cloves, crushed
- **1** tablespoon fresh rosemary leaves, minced
- **1** tablespoon fresh parsley leaves, minced
- Salt and ground black pepper, as required
- 4 (8-ounce) (1¼-inch-thick) lamb loin chops

For salad

- 4 cups fresh kale, tough ribs removed and torn
- **2** oranges, peeled and segmented
- **2** grapefruits, peeled and segmented
- 4 tablespoons unsweetened dried cranberries
- ½ teaspoon white sesame seeds

For Dressing

- 3 tablespoons extra-virgin olive oil
- 3 tablespoons fresh orange juice
- 2 teaspoons Dijon mustard
- 1 teaspoon raw honey
- Salt and ground black pepper, as required

Method:

1. In a large bowl, add **1** tablespoon extra- virgin olive oil, garlic, herbs, salt, and black pepper, and mix well.
2. Add the chops and coat with mixture generously.
3. Preheat oven to 400 degrees F.
4. cook the lamb chops for about 3 minutes per side in a heavy-bottomed skillet.
6. Bake chop in preheated oven for about **10** minutes.

7. Remove the lamb chops from the oven and place onto a platter.
8. Meanwhile, in a salad bowl, place all ingredients and mix.
9. Mix all ingredients in another bowl and beat until well combined.
10. Place dressing on top of salad and toss to coat well.
11. Divide the salad onto serving plates and top each with chops.
12. Serve immediately.

Flank Steak with Salad

Preparation time: 40 Min

Serves: 4

What you need:

For Steak

- **2** tablespoons extra-virgin olive oil
- 4 (6-ounce) flank steaks
- Salt and ground black pepper, as required

For Salad

- 6 cups fresh baby arugula
- **1** cup cherry tomatoes, halved
- **1** cup cucumber, chopped
- 3 tablespoons extra-virgin olive oil
- **2** tablespoons red wine vinegar
- Salt and ground black pepper, as required

Method:

1. Heat oil over medium-high heat and cook the steaks with salt and black pepper for about 4-5 minutes per side or until desired doneness.
2. Meanwhile, put all salad in a bowl and mix well.
3. Divide the arugula salad onto serving plates and top each with **1** steak.
4. Serve immediately.

Glazed Flank Steak

Preparation time: 40 Min

Serves: 4

What you need:

- **2** tablespoons arrowroot flour
- Salt and ground black pepper, as required
- **1½** pounds flank steak, cut into ¼-inch thick slices
- ½ cup extra-virgin olive oil, divided
- **1** onion, sliced
- **2** garlic cloves, minced
- **1** teaspoon fresh ginger, minced
- ¼ teaspoon red pepper flakes, crushed
- 1/3 cup raw honey
- ½ cup homemade beef broth
- ½ cup low-sodium soy sauce
- 5 tablespoons cashews
- **2** tablespoons fresh parsley, chopped

Method:

1. Mix arrowroot flour, salt, and black pepper in a bowl.
2. Coat the beef slices in arrowroot flour mixture evenly and then shake off excess mixture.
3. For sauce: In a pan, heat **1** tablespoon of oil over medium heat and sauté the onion for about 3-4 minutes.
4. Add garlic, ginger, and red pepper flakes and sauté for about **1** minute.
5. Add the honey, broth, and soy sauce and stir to combine well.
6. Increase the heat to high and cook for about 3 minutes, stirring continuously.
7. Remove the sauce from heat and set aside.

8. In a large sauté pan, heat the remaining oil over medium-high heat and fry the beef slices for about 3-4 minutes.
9. With a slotted spoon, transfer the beef slices onto a paper towel-lined plate to drain.
10. Remove the oil from the sauté pan, leaving about **1** tablespoon inside.
11. Return the beef slices into sauté pan over medium heat and sear the beef slices for about **2**-3 minutes.
12. Stir in honey sauce and cook for about 3-5 minutes.
13. Serve hot with the garnishing of cashews and parsley.

DESSERTS

Apple & Walnuts Cake

Preparation time: 50 Min

Serves: 16

What you need:

- 8 cups sliced peeled tart apples
- 1 cup dates syrup
- 2 cups walnuts milk
- 2 teaspoons ground cinnamon
- 1 cup walnut butter, softened
- 2 cups buckwheat flour
- 1 cup finely chopped walnuts, divided

Method:

1. Place apples in a greased 13x9-in baking dish.
2. Sprinkle with cinnamon.
3. Mix flour, milk, syrup, and walnuts in a bowl.
4. Pour mixture over apples. Sprinkle with remaining walnuts.
5. Bake at 350° for 45-55 minutes.
6. Serve and enjoy!

Per serving:

Calories Per **Serves:**, 293 kcal, 16.37 g Fat, 36.89 g Total Carbs, 3.89 g Protein, 3.3 g

Fiber

Baked Walnut Brownies

Preparation time: 30 Min

Serves: 16

What you need:
- 4 tablespoons walnuts butter
- 3/4 cup buckwheat flour
- 1/2 teaspoon salt
- 3/4 teaspoon baking powder
- 1/8 teaspoon baking soda
- 1 cup dates chopped
- ¼ cup dates syrup
- 1 cup walnuts (chopped)

Method:
1. Preheat oven to 350 F.
2. Grease brownies pan with cooking spray.
3. In a medium bowl, mix the dry ingredients until well incorporated.
4. Blend the dates, melted butter, dates, and walnuts in a blender.
5. Stir in flour mixture until well blended.
6. Pour the thick batter into the prepared baking pan and spread it evenly with a spatula.
7. Bake in the preheated oven for about 20 to 24 minutes, or until browned and the top has formed a crust.
8. Slice it.
9. Serve cold and enjoy!

Per serving:
Calories Per **Serves:**, 170 kcal, 6.57 g Fat, 27.85 g Total Carbs, 2.12 g Protein, 2.1 g Fiber

Coco & Walnuts Smoothie

Preparation time: 10 Min

Serves: 1

What you need:

- 1 cup soy milk
- 1 tsp dates syrup
- 1/2 oz. walnuts
- 1 tbsp. cocoa powder
- 1/2 cup ice cubes

Method:

1. Put all ingredients in a high-speed blender.
2. Blend until all ingredients are incorporated.
3. Serve and enjoy!

Per serving:

Calories Per **Serves:**, 262 kcal, 17.25 g Fat, 16.09 g Total Carbs, 9.85 g Protein, 1 g Fiber

Walnut Cream Cake

Preparation time: 40 Min

Serves: 10

What you need:
- 4 oz. buckwheat flour
- 1 teaspoon baking powder
- 4 oz. walnut cream
- ¼ cup dates syrup
- 1 cup soy milk
- 2 oz. walnut, chopped

Method:
1. Grease cake pan with cooking oil or olive oil
2. Mix the flour and baking powder, set aside.
3. Add dates syrup and the rest of the ingredients in the flour and mix well.
4. Pour the batter into the greased pan, shake gently to level off the batter.
5. Bake at a pre-heated oven at 180C (350F) for about 30-35 minutes or until cooked.
6. Serve and enjoy!

Per serving:
Calories Per **Serves:**, 195 kcal, 14.06 g Fat, 16.51 g Total Carbs, 3.16 g Protein, 1.5 g Fiber

Walnuts Bits

Preparation time: 40 Min

Serves: 20

What you need:

- 1/2 cup walnut butter softened
- 8 oz. walnut cream
- 1/2 cup dates, finely chopped
- 1 cup walnuts, chopped
- 1/2 cup dates, chopped
- 2 tbsps.sesame seeds

Method:

1. In a large bowl, mix all ingredients except chopped dates and sesame seeds.
2. Gently fold in chopped dates.
3. Use a cookie scoop to make 20 even bites and place onto prepared cookie sheet.
4. Roll on sesame seeds.
5. Place in fridge for 30 minutes - 1 hour, or until firm.
6. Serve and enjoy!

Per serving:

Calories Per **Serves:**, 185 kcal, 17.04 g Fat, 7.47 g Total Carbs, 2.92 g Protein, 1.9 g Fiber

Walnuts Bites Muffins

Preparation time: 40 Min

Serves: 12

What you need:
- 1/2 cup dates sugar
- 2 cups buckwheat flour
- 2 teaspoons baking powder
- 1/2 teaspoon salt
- 2/3 cup soy milk
- 1/2 cup walnut butter, melted, cooled
- 1 cup dark chocolate, melted
- 1/2 cup California walnuts, chopped

Method:
1. Preheat oven to 400°F. Grease or line 12 large muffin cups.
2. In a large bowl, mix sugars, buckwheat flour, baking powder, and salt. In a medium bowl, combine milk, butter, chocolate and blend well.
3. Mix dry ingredients with wet ingredients.
4. Pour batter into greased muffin cups.
5. Bake for 15 to 20 minutes or until cooked.
6. Serve hot and enjoy!

Per serving:
Calories Per **Serves:**, 271 kcal, 18.37 g Fat, 23.85 g Total Carbs, 5.51 g Protein, 4.7 g Fiber

Buckwheat Cinnamon Buns

Preparation time: 30 Min

Serves: 8

What you need:
- 14-16 oz. buckwheat dough
- 1 cup dates syrup
- 2 tbsps. cinnamon powder,
- 2 tbsps. walnut butter, melted

Method:
1. Preheat oven to 400 degrees F.
2. Roll dough into a rectangle about 10 X 14 inches.
3. Mix syrup and cinnamon powder in a mixing bowl.
4. Spread this mixture over rolled dough.
5. Roll dough in a circle.
6. Slice dough with knife or pizza cutter into 1-inch pieces. Place rolls on prepared sheets.
7. Quickly brush butter over rolls.
8. Bake rolls for about 15 minutes or until lightly brown and rolls are cooked through.

Per serving:
Calories Per **Serves:**, 170 kcal, 0.41 g Fat, 43.33 g Total Carbs, 1.8 g Protein, 1.4 g Fiber

Lightning Source UK Ltd.
Milton Keynes UK
UKHW020642160721
387267UK00011B/546